Fasting for Health: The Ultimate Guide to Transform Your Life

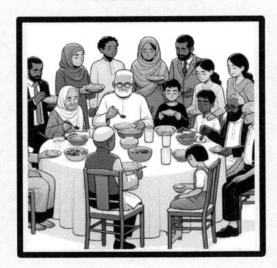

FASTING PIONEER

Fasting for Health: The Ultimate Guide to Transform Your Life

Fasting Pioneer

Published by Fasting Pioneer, 2024.

While every precaution has been taken in the preparation of this book, the publisher assumes no responsibility for errors or omissions, or for damages resulting from the use of the information contained herein.

FASTING FOR HEALTH: THE ULTIMATE GUIDE TO TRANSFORM YOUR LIFE

First edition. March 17, 2024.

Copyright © 2024 Fasting Pioneer.

Written by Fasting Pioneer.

To you, our readers,

This book is dedicated to anyone standing at the threshold of change, seeking a path to a healthier, more vibrant life. To the curious souls who dare to explore the transformative power of fasting, and to those who strive for wellness, not just for themselves but for the world around them.

We dedicate this journey to you, for your courage to embrace change, your willingness to learn, and your commitment to your health. May this guide be a beacon on your path to discovery, growth, and profound well-being.

With gratitude and hope,

The Fasting Pioneer Team

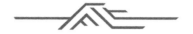

Chapter 1: The Basics of Fasting

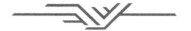

1.1: Understanding Fasting

Fasting is a practice that has been around for centuries and involves abstaining from food and, in some cases, drink for a specific period of time. It is not just a trend, but rather a practice deeply rooted in human history and various cultural and religious traditions. While the specific methods and reasons for fasting may vary, the underlying principle remains the same: the intentional withholding of food for spiritual, health, or therapeutic purposes.

There are several different types of fasting, each with its own unique approach and benefits. Intermittent fasting, for example, involves alternating periods of eating and fasting, typically on a daily basis. This method has gained popularity due to its potential to aid in weight loss, improve metabolic health, and reduce the risk of chronic diseases. On the other hand, prolonged or extended fasting typically lasts for 24 hours or more, and is believed to offer more profound health benefits such as cellular repair, autophagy, and improved insulin sensitivity.

Understanding the physiological effects of fasting can help shed light on its potential health benefits. When the body is deprived of food, it shifts into a state of ketosis, where it begins to burn fat for energy instead of glucose. This metabolic state has been associated with improved mental clarity, increased energy levels, and weight loss. Additionally, fasting triggers various hormonal responses, including the release of human growth hormone (HGH), which plays a role in muscle preservation, fat metabolism, and overall cellular repair.

Moreover, fasting has been linked to a wide range of potential health benefits, supported by scientific research. For instance, studies have suggested that intermittent fasting may reduce the risk of type 2 diabetes, heart disease, and certain types of cancer. It may also protect brain health, improve cognitive function, and enhance longevity. Furthermore, fasting has been shown to support the body's natural detoxification processes, promoting the elimination of toxins and waste products.

It is important to note that while fasting can offer numerous health benefits, it may not be suitable for everyone. Individuals with underlying medical conditions, pregnant or nursing women, and those with a history of disordered eating should exercise caution and consult with a healthcare professional before embarking on a fasting regimen. As with any lifestyle choice, it is crucial to approach fasting with mindfulness and a thorough understanding of its potential impact on individual health and well-being.

1.2: Different Types of Fasting

IN THE WORLD OF FASTING, there are various types that individuals can explore based on their health goals and preferences. Understanding the different types of fasting can help you make an informed decision about which approach may be best suited for you. One popular method is intermittent fasting, which involves cycling between periods of eating and fasting. The most common forms of intermittent fasting include the 16/8 method, where individuals fast for 16 hours and consume all their meals within an 8-hour window, and the 5:2 method, where individuals eat normally for five days of the week and restrict calorie intake on the remaining two days.

Another well-known fasting method is water fasting, which involves consuming only water for a designated period. This type of fasting is typically more challenging and should be approached with caution, as prolonged water fasting can lead to nutrient deficiencies and other health risks. On the other hand, juice fasting allows individuals to consume freshly squeezed fruit and vegetable juices for a set period, providing essential nutrients while still giving the digestive system a break.

Alternate-day fasting involves alternating between days of regular eating and fasting, which can take various forms such as complete fasting, consuming a limited amount of calories, or fasting with only specific foods or beverages allowed. Time-restricted feeding is another form of intermittent fasting that focuses on consuming all meals within a specific time frame each day.

Additionally, religious fasting practices such as Ramadan in Islam, Yom Kippur in Judaism, and Lent in Christianity also play a significant role in the lives of millions of people around the world. These fasting traditions often involve specific guidelines and time frames for abstinence from food and sometimes drink, serving as spiritual and cultural practices in addition to potential health benefits.

Beyond these common types, there are numerous other variations and hybrid approaches to fasting, each with its own unique set of guidelines and potential benefits. It's important to consider your individual health status, lifestyle, and goals when choosing a fasting method, and consulting with a healthcare professional before embarking on any fasting regimen is highly recommended. Understanding the various types of fasting empowers individuals to make informed choices that align with their personal needs and preferences, ultimately supporting their journey toward improved health and well-being.

1.3: Benefits of Fasting

IN THIS SECTION, WE will delve into the numerous benefits of fasting, providing valuable insights for parents, seniors, foodies, environmentalists, and travelers. Fasting has been shown to offer a wide range of health benefits, including weight loss, improved metabolic health, and enhanced heart health.

Intermittent fasting, in particular, has gained significant attention in recent years for its ability to aid weight loss and improve overall health.

Studies have shown that intermittent fasting can lead to a significant reduction in body weight and body fat percentage, which can have a positive impact on individuals looking to improve their overall health and well-being.

Furthermore, fasting has been linked to improved metabolic health, including better blood sugar control and insulin sensitivity. This can be particularly beneficial for individuals at risk of or managing type 2 diabetes. Research has indicated that intermittent fasting may lead to a decrease in insulin levels, which can help the body utilize insulin more effectively and improve blood sugar control.

In addition to these benefits, fasting has also been associated with improved heart health. Studies have suggested that fasting may lead to a reduction in risk factors for heart disease, including lower blood pressure, improved cholesterol levels, and a reduced likelihood of developing cardiovascular diseases. These findings underscore the potential of fasting as a tool for promoting heart health and reducing the risk of heart-related issues.

Moreover, fasting has been shown to have cognitive benefits, with research indicating that it may support brain health and function. Studies have found that fasting can stimulate the production of brain-derived neurotrophic factor (BDNF), a protein that supports the growth and maintenance of nerve cells. This could have implications for cognitive function, potentially contributing to improved brain health and a reduced risk of neurodegenerative conditions.

Beyond the physical and cognitive benefits, fasting also holds potential environmental and ethical advantages. By reducing the consumption of animal products and processed foods, individuals who practice fasting may contribute to a more sustainable and environmentally friendly food system. Additionally, some people choose to incorporate fasting as part of their lifestyle to align with ethical considerations related to food consumption and animal welfare.

Overall, the benefits of fasting are multifaceted, spanning from physical and metabolic health to cognitive well-being and ethical considerations. These potential advantages make fasting a compelling approach for individuals seeking to improve their health and make mindful choices about their dietary habits. As we continue to explore the topic of fasting, we will further examine the specific strategies and considerations for incorporating fasting into a balanced and healthy lifestyle.

1.4: Safety Considerations

WHEN EMBARKING ON A fasting journey, it is crucial to consider the safety aspects of this practice. While fasting can offer a wide array of health benefits, it is essential to approach it with caution, especially for specific demographic groups. For parents, seniors, foodies, environmentalists, and travelers, understanding the safety considerations of fasting is of utmost importance.

For individuals in the 30-50 age group, fasting can prove to be beneficial for weight management and overall health improvement. However, it is crucial to be aware of potential risks such as nutrient deficiencies and metabolic changes, particularly if there are underlying health conditions. Seniors (60+), who may be interested in fasting for its potential health benefits, should exercise greater caution due to age-related changes in metabolism and potential medication interactions. It is advisable for seniors to consult a healthcare professional before embarking on a fasting regimen to ensure that it is safe for their individual health status.

Foodies, who have a keen interest in culinary experiences and maintaining a healthy lifestyle, may find fasting intriguing. It is important for food enthusiasts to ensure that they approach fasting in a way that maintains adequate nutrient intake and does not lead to disordered eating patterns. Environmentalists, who are conscious about their impact on the planet, should consider sustainable fasting practices that do not compromise overall nutritional needs and contribute to food wastage. Travelers, who may have erratic schedules and dietary habits, should carefully plan fasting routines while considering the potential stressors of travel and the availability of nutrient-dense foods.

It is important to note that safety considerations for fasting also extend to specific medical conditions. Individuals with diabetes, hypoglycemia, eating disorders, or a history of disordered eating should approach fasting with caution or under the guidance of a healthcare professional. Pregnant or breastfeeding individuals should avoid fasting altogether due to the increased nutritional demands of these life stages.

It is essential to approach fasting with mindfulness and awareness of individual needs and circumstances. Understanding the potential risks and seeking guidance from healthcare professionals can significantly mitigate the likelihood of adverse effects. For anyone considering fasting, it's recommended to start with short fasting periods and gradually increase duration to allow the body to adapt. By being mindful of safety considerations, individuals can fully harness the benefits of fasting while prioritizing their health and well-being.

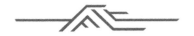

Chapter 2: Fasting and Nutrition

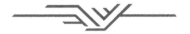

2.1: Nutritional Considerations During Fasting

When embarking on a fasting journey, it is crucial to consider the nutritional aspects to ensure that the body receives the essential nutrients it needs to function optimally. While fasting, the body undergoes various metabolic and hormonal changes, and it is important to support these changes with the right nutrition.

One of the most popular forms of fasting is intermittent fasting, where individuals cycle between periods of eating and fasting. During the eating windows, it is crucial to focus on consuming nutrient-dense foods to support overall health. These include fruits, vegetables, whole grains, lean proteins, and healthy fats. These foods provide essential vitamins, minerals, and antioxidants that are vital for the body's metabolic processes and overall well-being. It is essential to avoid processed foods, sugary snacks, and high-calorie beverages during the eating windows to maximize the benefits of fasting.

During extended fasts, such as water fasting or prolonged fasting, nutritional considerations become even more critical. It is highly recommended to consult a healthcare professional or a registered dietitian before undertaking prolonged fasting to ensure that the body's nutritional needs are met. While fasting, the body relies on stored nutrients for energy, and it is important to ensure that the body has an adequate supply of essential vitamins and minerals. Electrolyte imbalances can occur during prolonged fasting, leading to symptoms such as fatigue, dizziness, and muscle cramps. Therefore, it is important to consider supplementing with electrolytes or consuming bone broths to replenish essential minerals such as sodium, potassium, and magnesium.

It is also essential to stay well-hydrated during fasting periods. Water is crucial for maintaining cellular function, regulating body temperature, and supporting the body's natural detoxification processes. Herbal teas and black coffee can also be consumed during fasting periods, but it is important to avoid adding sugar or cream to these beverages, as they can break the fast and spike insulin levels.

For parents, seniors, foodies, environmentalists, and travelers engaging in fasting, it is important to plan meals and fasting periods that align with their lifestyle and dietary preferences. Parents may need to consider the nutritional needs of their children while fasting, ensuring that their family's meals are balanced and nourishing. Seniors should be mindful of their individual health conditions and medications while fasting, seeking guidance from healthcare professionals when necessary. Foodies may explore creative and nutritious meal options for their eating windows, making the fasting experience enjoyable and sustainable. Environmentalists may consider the environmental impact of their food choices during eating windows, opting for sustainable and ethically sourced ingredients. Travelers may need to plan ahead to ensure that they have access to nutritious foods and beverages during fasting periods while on the go.

In conclusion, nutritional considerations during fasting are pivotal for maintaining overall health and well-being. Whether engaging in intermittent fasting or prolonged fasting, prioritizing nutrient-dense foods, staying hydrated, and seeking professional guidance when needed are essential for a safe and effective fasting experience. By incorporating these nutritional considerations, individuals can harness the full benefits of fasting and optimize their health outcomes.

2.2: Fasting and Weight Management

INCORPORATING FASTING into your lifestyle can be an effective strategy for managing weight. Fasting helps to reduce calorie intake and promote weight loss by putting the body in a state of ketosis, where it starts burning fat for energy. A study published in JAMA Internal Medicine found that intermittent fasting can lead to significant weight loss, with participants losing an average of 7-11 pounds over a period of 10 weeks. Another study conducted by the University of Illinois at Chicago reported that alternate day fasting resulted in an average weight loss of 12 pounds over a 12-week period. These findings suggest that fasting can be an impactful tool for weight management.

Fasting also influences hormone levels that are involved in weight regulation. For example, during fasting, insulin levels decrease, which promotes fat burning. Additionally, growth hormone levels increase during fasting, aiding in the preservation of muscle mass while promoting fat loss. Furthermore, fasting has been shown to positively impact the body's metabolic rate. A study published in the American Journal of Clinical Nutrition demonstrated that alternate day fasting can increase metabolic rate by up to 14%, contributing to more efficient calorie burning.

It's important to note that while fasting can be an effective tool for weight management, it should be approached with caution and under the guidance of a healthcare professional, especially for individuals with underlying health conditions. Fasting has the potential to lead to nutrient deficiencies if not properly planned, and may not be suitable for everyone. It's essential to ensure that nutritional needs are met during non-fasting periods to support overall health and well-being. Additionally, fasting may not be suitable for individuals with a history of disordered eating or certain medical conditions, so it's crucial to consult with a healthcare provider before embarking on a fasting regimen.

In summary, fasting can be a valuable approach for weight management, promoting weight loss, influencing hormone levels, and positively impacting metabolic rate. However, it's important to approach fasting with caution and seek professional guidance to ensure that it is done in a safe and sustainable manner. By integrating fasting into a well-rounded approach to nutrition and lifestyle, individuals can harness its potential benefits for weight management and overall health.

2.3: Fasting for Mental Clarity

FASTING IS NOT JUST about physical health; it also has numerous benefits for our mental well-being. One of the most remarkable benefits of fasting is its potential to enhance mental clarity. With various fasting methods, such as intermittent fasting and time-restricted eating, individuals report improved focus, concentration, and cognitive function. Research has shown that fasting can stimulate the production of brain-derived neurotrophic factor (BDNF), a protein that supports the growth and maintenance of neurons, as well as the development of new synapses. The increase in BDNF levels during fasting has been linked to enhanced cognitive function, learning, and memory retention.

Furthermore, fasting has been found to regulate the levels of neurotransmitters such as dopamine and serotonin, which are crucial for mood regulation and mental well-being. By promoting a balance in these neurotransmitters, fasting may contribute to reducing symptoms of anxiety and depression and improving overall mental clarity. Studies have demonstrated that fasting can also reduce inflammation in the brain, which is associated with cognitive decline and neurodegenerative diseases. This anti-inflammatory effect may further contribute to improved mental clarity and sharpness.

In addition, fasting has been shown to promote autophagy, a cellular cleansing process that eliminates damaged cells and organelles. This cellular "spring cleaning" not only supports overall physical health but also has implications for mental clarity and cognitive function. With the removal of cellular waste and toxins, the brain may function more efficiently, leading to heightened mental acuity and clarity. Moreover, fasting can influence the gut-brain axis, the bidirectional communication pathway between the gut and the brain. The balance of gut microbiota, which can be positively impacted by fasting, plays a crucial role in mental health, with studies suggesting a link between gut dysbiosis and conditions such as anxiety and depression.

It's important to note that individual experiences with fasting and mental clarity may vary, and consulting with a healthcare professional is essential, especially for individuals with pre-existing medical conditions or those taking medications. While many people report mental clarity benefits from fasting, it's crucial to approach fasting with mindfulness and listen to your body's signals. As with any dietary or lifestyle change, it's wise to start gradually and monitor how your body and mind respond to fasting practices.

In conclusion, the potential for fasting to enhance mental clarity is an intriguing aspect of its broader health benefits. The impact of fasting on brain function, neurotransmitter regulation, inflammation reduction, and cellular cleansing suggests that fasting can be a powerful tool for improving cognitive function and mental well-being. As further research continues to investigate the relationship between fasting and mental clarity, it is essential to approach fasting as part of a holistic approach to health, encompassing nutrition, physical activity, and overall well-being.

2.4: Fasting for Physical Performance

INCORPORATING FASTING into your lifestyle can have significant effects on physical performance. While many people may worry about feeling weak or fatigued during a fast, research shows that fasting can actually improve physical performance by enhancing metabolism and increasing energy levels. During fasting, the body shifts from using glucose for energy to utilizing stored fat, leading to more sustainable and steady energy levels. This process, known as metabolic switching, can greatly benefit athletes and fitness enthusiasts by improving endurance and stamina. Studies have demonstrated that intermittent fasting can promote fat oxidation and enhance exercise performance. For example, a study published in the Journal of the International Society of Sports Nutrition found that intermittent fasting led to improvements in body composition and enhanced endurance performance in athletes.

Furthermore, fasting can contribute to overall fitness and muscle preservation.

While fasting, the body produces higher levels of growth hormone, which plays a crucial role in muscle growth, fat metabolism, and maintenance of lean body mass. Research suggests that short-term fasting can increase growth hormone secretion, thus promoting muscle preservation and supporting physical performance. Additionally, fasting has been shown to have anti-inflammatory effects, which can aid in faster recovery after intense workouts or physical activities. By reducing inflammation and enhancing cellular repair processes, fasting can support the body's resilience to physical stress and improve overall performance.

It's important to note that fasting for physical performance should be approached with caution and individualized based on personal health conditions and fitness goals. Consulting with a healthcare professional or nutritionist is crucial to ensure that fasting is implemented safely and effectively. For athletes or individuals with specific training regimens, it's essential to carefully plan fasting periods around workout schedules and ensure adequate nutrient intake during non-fasting periods. Ensuring proper hydration and consuming balanced meals when breaking a fast is essential for optimizing physical performance and recovery.

In conclusion, fasting can be a beneficial strategy for improving physical performance, enhancing metabolism, and supporting overall fitness. Incorporating intermittent fasting into your routine can lead to metabolic adaptations that promote fat oxidation, endurance, and muscle preservation. However, it's essential to approach fasting for physical performance with careful consideration of individual health and fitness needs and to seek professional guidance when implementing fasting practices. By doing so, you can unlock the potential benefits of fasting to support and enhance your physical performance and overall well-being.

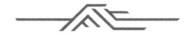

Chapter 3: Fasting and Age

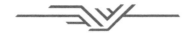

3.1: Fasting for Parents (30-50)

In today's fast-paced world, parents in the age range of 30-50 often find themselves juggling careers, family responsibilities, and various other commitments. As a result, maintaining a healthy lifestyle can sometimes take a backseat. However, implementing fasting into their routine can offer numerous health benefits that can positively impact their overall well-being.

Fasting has been shown to be particularly beneficial for parents in this age group as it can aid in weight management, improve metabolic health, and reduce the risk of chronic diseases. Research has indicated that intermittent fasting, which involves cycling between periods of eating and fasting, can lead to significant weight loss and a reduction in visceral fat, particularly in individuals in the 30-50 age bracket (Ganesan, Arumugam, & Guizani, 2018). Furthermore, it can contribute to improved insulin sensitivity and reduced inflammation, both of which are crucial for maintaining optimal health in this age group.

For parents, fasting can also promote mental clarity and enhance cognitive function, which can be invaluable when balancing the demands of work and family life. Studies have suggested that intermittent fasting may have neuroprotective effects and could potentially reduce the risk of neurodegenerative diseases such as Alzheimer's and Parkinson's (Mattson, Moehl, & Ghena, 2014). This aspect of fasting is particularly relevant for individuals in the 30-50 age group, as it can help sustain mental acuity and cognitive sharpness during this pivotal stage of life.

Moreover, implementing a fasting regimen can have a positive impact on aging-related markers, potentially slowing down the aging process and promoting longevity. Research has shown that fasting can stimulate cellular repair processes and enhance the body's ability to combat oxidative stress, which is especially relevant for individuals in the 30-50 age range as it can aid in mitigating the effects of aging on the body (Longo & Mattson, 2014). These agerelated benefits of fasting can be particularly appealing to parents who are looking to maintain their vitality and vigor as they navigate the responsibilities of both parenthood and career.

In conclusion, fasting can be a powerful tool for parents in the 30-50 age group to optimize their health and well-being. By incorporating fasting into their lifestyle, parents can potentially experience improvements in weight management, metabolic health, cognitive function, and aging-related markers. As they strive to balance the demands of parenthood, career, and personal wellness, integrating fasting as a health strategy can offer a multitude of benefits to support their overall vitality and longevity.

3.2: Fasting for Seniors (60+)

AS WE AGE, OUR BODIES undergo various changes, and it is essential to consider how fasting can affect seniors (60+). Fasting for seniors can offer numerous health benefits but also requires careful consideration and monitoring. Research has shown that fasting can help improve cardiovascular health, reduce inflammation, and regulate blood sugar levels, all of which are particularly important for seniors. However, it's crucial for seniors to approach fasting with caution and consult with a healthcare professional before making any significant changes to their eating patterns.

One significant benefit of fasting for seniors is its potential to improve cognitive function. Studies have shown that intermittent fasting may help protect against age-related cognitive decline and neurodegenerative diseases such as Alzheimer's and Parkinson's. As we age, brain function becomes increasingly important, and the potential cognitive benefits of fasting are compelling.

Additionally, fasting has been linked to increased longevity and a reduced risk of age-related diseases. A study published in Cell Metabolism found that periodic fasting in mice led to an increase in lifespan and a decrease in the incidence of age-related diseases. While more research is needed to fully understand the effects of fasting on human longevity, these initial findings are promising.

It's important to note that seniors may have unique considerations when it comes to fasting. For example, many seniors take multiple medications, and fasting can potentially affect the way these medications are absorbed and metabolized in the body. Seniors may also be more susceptible to dehydration, so it's essential for them to stay well-hydrated and monitor their fluid intake carefully during fasting periods.

Another consideration for seniors is the potential impact of fasting on muscle mass and bone density. As we age, preserving muscle mass and bone density becomes increasingly important for overall health and mobility. Research suggests that incorporating resistance training and maintaining adequate protein intake can help mitigate the potential loss of muscle and bone mass associated with fasting.

In conclusion, fasting can offer various health benefits for seniors, including improved cardiovascular health, cognitive function, and longevity. However, it's crucial for seniors to approach fasting with caution, consult with a healthcare professional, and consider their unique health needs and circumstances. With careful consideration and monitoring, seniors can potentially reap the benefits of fasting while maintaining their overall health and well-being.

3.3: Adapting Fasting to Different Life Stages

INCORPORATING FASTING into your lifestyle is a powerful tool for optimizing health at any age, but it's important to consider how to adapt fasting to different life stages. As we age, our nutritional needs and metabolic functions change, and it's crucial to understand how fasting can be modified to accommodate these changes.

For parents in the 30-50 age range, incorporating fasting can offer numerous health benefits. Research has shown that intermittent fasting may aid in weight management, reduce the risk of chronic diseases, and improve metabolic health. However, it's important for parents to approach fasting with caution and take into account their busy schedules and energy requirements for caring for their families. For parents in this age group, a time-restricted eating (TRE) approach, such as the 16/8 method (fasting for 16 hours and eating within an 8hour window), can be a practical and effective way to reap the benefits of fasting while still meeting their nutritional needs and energy demands.

Seniors aged 60 and above often face age-related health challenges and changes in nutrient absorption and metabolism. When considering fasting, it's crucial for seniors to consult with a healthcare professional to ensure that fasting is safe and appropriate for their individual health status. A modified fasting approach, such as the 5:2 method (eating regularly for five days and consuming fewer calories on two non-consecutive days), may be more suitable for seniors, as it allows for flexibility and may provide the health benefits of fasting without being overly restrictive. Additionally, older adults should prioritize nutrient-dense foods and adequate hydration during fasting periods to support their overall health and well-being.

Foodies who have a passion for culinary experiences may find fasting to be a transformative addition to their lifestyle. Fasting can enhance appreciation for food and flavors, promote mindful eating, and provide an opportunity to explore new recipes and cooking techniques. Intermittent fasting, combined with a focus on high-quality, nutrient-rich foods during eating periods, can complement a foodie's love for gastronomy while supporting metabolic health and wellbeing.

Environmentalists who are dedicated to sustainability and mindful consumption can integrate fasting into their lifestyle as a way to minimize food waste and reduce their environmental footprint. By embracing meal planning and conscious food choices during eating periods, individuals with an environmental focus can contribute to reducing the impact of food production and consumption on the environment while simultaneously reaping the health benefits of fasting.

Travelers who frequently find themselves on the go can also explore the adaptability of fasting to different time zones and travel schedules. Fasting can offer a practical and flexible approach to nutrition while traveling, allowing individuals to maintain their health and well-being even in unfamiliar surroundings. Fasting may help mitigate the challenges of jet lag, irregular meal times, and exposure to new cuisines, providing travelers with a sense of control over their nutrition and overall health during their adventures.

3.4: Managing Fasting with Age-related Concerns

INCORPORATING FASTING into your lifestyle can have unique implications as you age. Regardless of your age, it's important to consult with a healthcare professional before initiating any fasting regimen, particularly if you have pre-existing health conditions. For seniors in particular, fasting may require more careful management due to the potential impact on medication schedules, nutrient requirements, and overall health. As we age, our bodies undergo various physiological changes, such as a decline in metabolic rate and potentially decreased muscle mass. These changes can influence how fasting might affect older individuals compared to younger adults.

One important consideration for seniors engaging in fasting is the potential impact on medication usage. Many seniors take prescription medications to manage various health conditions, and fasting can alter how these medications are absorbed and metabolized in the body. It's crucial for seniors to work closely with their healthcare providers to adjust medication schedules as needed to ensure safety and efficacy. Additionally, the potential for nutrient deficiencies is a concern for seniors when fasting. As we age, our bodies may have decreased nutrient absorption and increased nutrient requirements. Fasting could exacerbate these issues, potentially leading to deficiencies in essential vitamins and minerals. Tailoring a fasting plan that addresses these concerns, perhaps through nutrient-dense meal choices or supplementation, is crucial for seniors.

Furthermore, older individuals may need to be mindful of their muscle mass and overall physical health when considering fasting. Sarcopenia, the age-related loss of muscle mass and strength, can impact older adults' ability to withstand prolonged periods of fasting. It's important for seniors to maintain physical activity and muscle-strengthening exercises to mitigate the effects of sarcopenia while incorporating fasting into their lifestyle. Research has shown that intermittent fasting in combination with resistance training can help preserve muscle mass in older adults, emphasizing the importance of a holistic approach to managing fasting with age-related concerns.

For parents in the 30-50 age group, fasting can also present unique considerations. Balancing the demands of parenting with fasting may require careful planning and consideration of family meal dynamics. Intermittent fasting, for example, may need to be structured around family mealtimes and activities to ensure it aligns with the household's needs and routines. Additionally, for individuals within this age range, the potential impact of fasting on energy levels and mental acuity during busy parenting duties is a factor to bear in mind. It's essential for parents to assess how fasting may impact their ability to fulfill parental responsibilities and address any concerns with a healthcare professional if necessary.

Foodies and travelers, regardless of age, may find fasting to be a rewarding yet challenging endeavor. Exploring different cuisines and dining experiences can be a central aspect of their hobbies and travels. Introducing fasting into these activities may necessitate a shift in mindset and planning. For foodies, fasting could provide an opportunity to deepen their appreciation for culinary experiences and explore the cultural and historical significance of fasting practices in different regions. Meanwhile, travelers may need to carefully plan their fasting schedules around their journeys, considering factors such as time zone changes and access to suitable food options during fasting periods. Adapting fasting practices to align with the enjoyment of food and travel experiences can be a fulfilling but complex endeavor, requiring flexibility and creativity.

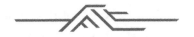

Chapter 4: Fasting and Lifestyle

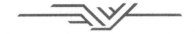

4.1: Fasting for Foodies

For foodies who are passionate about culinary experiences, the idea of fasting may initially seem daunting or even unappealing. However, integrating fasting into a foodie lifestyle can actually lead to a deeper appreciation for food and an enhanced sensory experience. By taking periodic breaks from eating, foodies can allow their taste buds to reset and their palate to become more sensitive to flavors, ultimately enhancing the enjoyment of meals. Additionally, fasting can also promote mindfulness around food, encouraging foodies to savor and fully experience each bite when they do eat.

Intermittent fasting, in particular, has gained popularity among foodies for its potential health benefits while still allowing for enjoyment of a wide variety of foods. Research has shown that intermittent fasting can lead to improvements in metabolic health, such as increased insulin sensitivity and reduced inflammation, which are important factors for foodies looking to maintain optimal health while indulging in diverse culinary delights. Intermittent fasting can also provide foodies with an opportunity to explore new recipes and cooking techniques during periods of fasting, fostering creativity and innovation in the kitchen.

Moreover, intermittent fasting can be seamlessly integrated into various foodie lifestyles, whether they revolve around exploring local cuisines, indulging in gourmet dining experiences, or experimenting with home cooking. Foodies who are frequent travelers can benefit from intermittent fasting as a practical way to adapt to different time zones and dining schedules while minimizing digestive discomfort. As for environmentalists, embracing intermittent fasting can align with their commitment to sustainable food practices by promoting mindful consumption and reducing food waste.

When it comes to seniors, intermittent fasting has shown promise in promoting healthy aging and longevity. Studies have demonstrated that intermittent fasting can enhance cellular repair processes, improve cognitive function, and reduce the risk of age-related chronic diseases, offering seniors an effective means to maintain vitality and well-being in their later years. Additionally, intermittent fasting may also support seniors in managing age-related changes in metabolism and body composition, contributing to a higher quality of life.

For parents in the 30-50 age range, integrating fasting into their busy lifestyles can present unique opportunities to prioritize their health and well-being. Many parents juggle multiple responsibilities and may find it challenging to make time for healthy eating habits. Intermittent fasting can offer a flexible approach that accommodates their hectic schedules while still allowing for enjoyment of family meals and bonding over food. By adopting intermittent fasting, parents can role model positive eating behaviors for their children and instill healthy attitudes towards food and nutrition from an early age. Furthermore, intermittent fasting can aid parents in managing weight and promoting metabolic health, which are crucial considerations for maintaining energy levels and overall vitality while raising a family.

In conclusion, fasting can be a valuable and enriching practice for foodies, seniors, parents, and individuals with a deep appreciation for diverse culinary experiences. By embracing intermittent fasting as a complementary lifestyle choice, individuals in these demographic groups can enhance their relationship with food, prioritize their health, and cultivate a greater sense of well-being.

4.2: Fasting for Environmentalists

FOR ENVIRONMENTALISTS, fasting can also be seen as a sustainable lifestyle choice that promotes eco-friendly living. The industrial food system, with its reliance on factory farming, has been linked to significant environmental issues such as deforestation, water pollution, and greenhouse gas emissions. By adopting a fasting lifestyle, environmentalists can minimize their ecological footprint and support sustainable food practices.

A key environmental benefit of fasting is the reduction of meat consumption. Livestock production accounts for a significant portion of global greenhouse gas emissions, with one study estimating that 14.5% of all anthropogenic greenhouse gas emissions are attributable to livestock. By incorporating fasting periods that focus on plant-based nutrition, individuals can significantly reduce their carbon footprint and contribute to mitigating climate change. Moreover, reducing meat consumption through fasting can also help conserve water, as the production of meat is more water-intensive compared to plant-based foods.

Fasting can also lead to reduced food waste, another pressing environmental concern. In the United States alone, it is estimated that around 30-40% of the food supply is wasted, leading to increased methane emissions in landfills and unnecessary strain on natural resources. By adopting a mindful approach to eating through fasting, individuals can become more conscious of food consumption and minimize food waste, thereby contributing to conservation efforts and reducing environmental impact.

Furthermore, fasting can encourage individuals to support local and sustainable food sources. By being more intentional about the quality and sourcing of their food during non-fasting periods, environmentalists can promote agricultural practices that prioritize biodiversity, soil health, and reduced chemical inputs. This, in turn, supports local farmers and promotes a more resilient and sustainable food system.

In addition to dietary aspects, incorporating fasting into one's lifestyle can also extend to reducing energy consumption. As fasting often involves simplifying meals and reducing reliance on processed and packaged foods, it can lead to a decrease in the energy and resources required for food production, processing, and transportation. This aligns with the principles of environmental sustainability and can contribute to overall efforts to reduce the ecological impact of the food industry.

Ultimately, fasting for environmentalists can be a holistic practice that extends beyond personal health benefits to encompass wider environmental stewardship. By making conscious choices about food consumption, waste reduction, and support for sustainable food systems, individuals can align their fasting lifestyle with their commitment to environmental conservation and sustainable living.

In conclusion, fasting offers a range of environmental benefits that can resonate with the values and principles of environmentalists. By reducing meat consumption, minimizing food waste, supporting local and sustainable food sources, and decreasing energy consumption, fasting can become a powerful tool for promoting ecological sustainability and contributing to a healthier planet for present and future generations.

4.3: Fasting for Travelers

FASTING FOR TRAVELERS can be a unique challenge, but with proper planning and mindfulness, it can also be a rewarding experience. Whether you are embarking on a short trip or a longer journey, incorporating fasting into your travel routine can have numerous benefits for your body and mind. One of the key advantages of fasting while traveling is the potential for reduced jet lag. Studies have shown that fasting can help reset the body's internal clock and ease the symptoms of jet lag, allowing travelers to adjust to new time zones more easily. Additionally, fasting can contribute to increased mental clarity and focus, which can be especially beneficial when navigating unfamiliar destinations or handling travel-related stressors.

When fasting during travel, it's important to consider the potential challenges and make adjustments accordingly. For instance, access to suitable food options may be limited, particularly in transit or in foreign locations. Planning ahead and packing nutritious, non-perishable snacks can help ensure that you have sustenance readily available during periods of fasting. It is also essential to stay well-hydrated while traveling, especially when fasting, as dehydration can exacerbate the effects of travel fatigue and disrupt the body's natural rhythms. Opting for water or herbal teas during fasting periods can support hydration and promote overall well-being.

Intermittent fasting, which involves cycling between periods of eating and fasting, can be particularly well-suited for travelers. By structuring fasting periods around travel plans, individuals can mitigate potential disruptions to their routine and optimize the fasting experience. For example, if you have a long flight or train journey ahead, planning a fasting period during the duration of the trip can help you stay energized and comfortable while minimizing the need for in-flight or on-the-go meals, which may not always align with your dietary preferences or restrictions.

It's essential to approach fasting for travel with flexibility and mindfulness, especially when exploring new culinary experiences. While fasting can enhance mindfulness and appreciation for food, it's also important to respect and honor local food traditions and customs. Engaging in research ahead of time to identify fasting-friendly options or cultural practices related to fasting in your travel destination can provide valuable insight and enrich your overall travel experience.

Fasting can be a powerful tool for maintaining health and well-being while on the road. By incorporating fasting into your travel lifestyle, you can optimize your body's resilience, adaptability, and vitality, allowing you to fully embrace the enriching experiences that travel has to offer.

4.4: Incorporating Fasting into Daily Routine

INCORPORATING FASTING into your daily routine can be a powerful way to enhance your overall health and well-being. By strategically implementing fasting periods into your lifestyle, you can optimize your body's natural healing processes, regulate your metabolism, and improve your mental clarity. As a busy parent, senior, foodie, environmentalist, or traveler, finding ways to seamlessly integrate fasting into your daily routine can seem daunting, but with careful planning and a bit of creativity, you can easily achieve this.

One of the most common and practical ways to incorporate fasting into your daily routine is through time-restricted eating, such as the popular 16/8 method.

This approach involves fasting for 16 hours and restricting your eating window to 8 hours each day. For example, you may choose to skip breakfast and consume your first meal around noon, then finish your last meal by 8 pm. This allows you to reap the benefits of fasting without drastically altering your daily schedule. Research has shown that time-restricted eating can help improve metabolic health, reduce inflammation, and support weight management. In fact, a study published in the journal Cell Metabolism found that restricting eating to an 8- to 10-hour window resulted in significant reductions in body weight, blood pressure, and cholesterol levels for participants with obesity.

Another effective way to integrate fasting into your lifestyle is by incorporating periodic fasting into your weekly or monthly routine. This can be achieved through methods such as the 5:2 diet, which involves consuming a limited number of calories (around 500-600) on two nonconsecutive days of the week while eating normally on the remaining days. For instance, you might choose to fast on Mondays and Thursdays while maintaining your regular eating pattern on the other five days. Studies have demonstrated that intermittent fasting, including the 5:2 approach, can lead to improvements in insulin sensitivity, cardiovascular health, and cellular repair processes. Additionally, intermittent fasting has been associated with a decrease in markers of inflammation and a reduction in the risk of chronic diseases such as diabetes and heart disease.

For travelers and individuals with dynamic schedules, fasting can be seamlessly integrated into daily life by planning ahead and making mindful choices.

Packing nutritious, low-calorie snacks for travel days can support intermittent fasting while on the go. Similarly, incorporating leisurely walks or light physical activity during fasting periods can help mitigate hunger pangs and promote fat utilization for energy. Furthermore, being mindful of hydration and consuming ample water, herbal teas, and broths during fasting periods can aid in maintaining energy levels and supporting overall well-being.

Incorporating fasting into your daily routine can be a transformative and empowering experience, regardless of your lifestyle or age. By embracing strategic fasting practices, you can optimize your health, support environmental sustainability, and enhance your overall quality of life. Whether you choose to implement a time-restricted eating schedule, periodic fasting approach, or make conscious decisions during travel, the benefits of fasting are accessible and adaptable to your unique daily routine, setting the stage for a healthier and more fulfilling lifestyle.

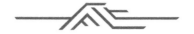

Chapter 5: Fasting Protocols

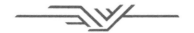

5.1: Intermittent Fasting

Intermittent fasting (IF) has gained significant popularity in recent years as a dietary approach that involves cycling between periods of eating and fasting. While intermittent fasting has been practiced for centuries, its potential health benefits have sparked a surge of interest and research. IF offers various protocols, but the most common ones include the 16/8 method, the 5:2 diet, and alternate-day fasting.

The 16/8 method, also known as the Leangains protocol, involves fasting for 16 hours and restricting your daily eating period to 8 hours. This can be easily implemented by skipping breakfast and consuming all meals within the remaining 8-hour window. The 5:2 diet, on the other hand, allows for unrestricted eating for five days a week and restricts caloric intake to 500-600 calories on the remaining two non-consecutive days. Lastly, alternate-day fasting involves alternating between eating normally one day and fasting the next. These diverse approaches provide flexibility, making intermittent fasting adaptable to different lifestyles.

Research has shown that intermittent fasting may offer numerous health benefits. One study published in the New England Journal of Medicine found that intermittent fasting can lead to weight loss and improvements in biomarkers associated with cardiovascular health. Another study in the journal Cell Metabolism reported that IF can enhance metabolic health by reducing insulin resistance and lowering the risk of type 2 diabetes. Furthermore, intermittent fasting has been linked to improved brain health, as it may enhance cognitive function and protect against age-related neurodegenerative diseases.

In addition to the potential health benefits, intermittent fasting can also promote sustainable living and environmental consciousness. By consuming fewer meals, individuals practicing intermittent fasting may reduce their overall food consumption, leading to decreased food waste and a lighter environmental footprint. Moreover, the simplicity of some IF protocols can appeal to travelers and foodies, as it offers a flexible approach to eating that aligns with diverse culinary experiences and lifestyles.

When considering intermittent fasting, it's crucial to consult with a healthcare professional, especially for seniors and parents. While intermittent fasting can be safe and effective for many individuals, it may not be suitable for everyone, particularly those with certain medical conditions or nutritional needs. Additionally, it's important to maintain balanced nutrition during eating periods to ensure that the body receives essential nutrients and energy. Overall, intermittent fasting presents a compelling approach to dietary patterns and offers potential benefits for individuals seeking to enhance their health and wellbeing.

In conclusion, intermittent fasting encompasses various protocols that can be tailored to fit different age groups and lifestyles, including parents, seniors, foodies, environmentalists, and travelers. The flexibility of IF, coupled with its potential health benefits and its promotion of sustainable living, makes it a noteworthy dietary approach worth considering for those seeking to transform their lives through fasting.

5.2: Extended Fasting

IN THE REALM OF FASTING protocols, extended fasting represents a more intensive approach that involves abstaining from food for an extended period, typically lasting 24 hours or longer. This practice has garnered attention for its potential health benefits, including weight loss, improved metabolic function, cellular repair, and mental clarity. It's important to note that extended fasting should be undertaken with caution and under the guidance of a healthcare professional, particularly for in-

dividuals with underlying health conditions or those who are pregnant or breastfeeding.

Research has shown that extended fasting can lead to significant changes in the body's hormone levels, including reduced insulin and increased growth hormone secretion, which may contribute to enhanced fat burning and muscle preservation. Moreover, studies have demonstrated that prolonged fasting can trigger autophagy, a process in which the body cleans out damaged cells and regenerates new ones, thereby promoting overall cellular health and potentially reducing the risk of certain chronic diseases.

It's worth noting that extended fasting is not suitable for everyone, and individual responses to this practice can vary widely. Seniors (60+) and individuals with existing health concerns should exercise particular caution and consult with a healthcare provider before embarking on an extended fast. Furthermore, extended fasting may not be ideal for parents (30-50) who are actively involved in caring for young children or for those who engage in intense physical activity on a regular basis.

For foodies who are considering extended fasting, it's important to approach this practice with mindfulness and a focus on nourishing the body with nutrient-dense foods before and after the fasting period. Prioritizing hydration and consuming adequate electrolytes can also be crucial during extended fasting to support overall well-being. Additionally, environmentalists and travelers may find extended fasting to be a convenient and sustainable approach to nutrition, especially when access to food options is limited.

Ultimately, while extended fasting holds potential benefits for certain individuals, it's essential to weigh the risks and benefits carefully and consider seeking guidance from a qualified healthcare professional. As with any fasting protocol, it's crucial to listen to your body and prioritize overall health and well-being throughout the process.

5.3: Fasting Mimicking Diet

IN THE REALM OF FASTING protocols, the Fasting Mimicking Diet (FMD) has gained significant attention for its potential health benefits. The Fasting Mimicking Diet was developed by Prof. Valter Longo, and it is a carefully designed meal plan that aims to provide the benefits of a prolonged fast while still allowing the consumption of some food. This approach combines a low-calorie, plant-based diet with precise amounts of macro and micronutrients to mimic the effects of fasting on the body without abstaining from food entirely. The Fasting Mimicking Diet typically lasts for 5 consecutive days and is then followed by a period of normal eating. During the fasting days, the diet restricts daily caloric intake to approximately 40-50% of normal intake, with specific ratios of protein, fats, and carbohydrates.

One of the primary potential benefits of the Fasting Mimicking Diet is its ability to promote cellular rejuvenation, a process known as autophagy. Autophagy is a cellular self-cleansing mechanism that removes damaged components and helps the body regenerate healthier cells. Consequently, this process has been linked to various health benefits, including improved metabolic health, reduced inflammation, and enhanced longevity. Additionally, research on the Fasting Mimicking Diet has revealed promising outcomes in terms of weight management, cardiovascular health, and metabolic function. Studies have demonstrated that participants following the Fasting Mimicking Diet experienced reductions in body weight, abdominal fat, blood glucose levels, and other risk factors associated with chronic diseases.

Furthermore, the Fasting Mimicking Diet has been suggested to have potential applications in the treatment and prevention of certain health conditions. Clinical studies have shown positive effects of the Fasting Mimicking Diet on conditions such as multiple sclerosis, cancer, and aging-related cognitive decline. Moreover, the Fasting Mimicking Diet has been associated with improved markers of overall health, such as cholesterol levels, blood pressure, and insulin sensitivity. These findings indicate that the Fasting Mimicking Diet has the potential to be a valuable tool in promoting overall well-being and improving health outcomes for individuals across different age groups and health statuses.

For parents, seniors, foodies, environmentalists, and travelers interested in exploring the Fasting Mimicking Diet, it is essential to approach it with caution and seek guidance from healthcare professionals, especially if they have existing medical conditions or are taking medications. While the potential health benefits of the Fasting Mimicking Diet are compelling, it is crucial to consider individual health circumstances and nutritional needs before embarking on such a dietary intervention. Additionally, incorporating the Fasting Mimicking Diet into a lifestyle that aligns with personal values and preferences, such as sustainability and ethical food choices, can enhance the overall experience and adherence to the protocol.

In conclusion, the Fasting Mimicking Diet represents an innovative approach to fasting that offers several potential health benefits, including cellular rejuvenation, weight management, and metabolic improvements. As ongoing research continues to unveil the mechanisms and applications of the Fasting Mimicking Diet, it holds promise as a valuable tool for optimizing health and wellbeing. While it presents exciting opportunities for individuals across various demographics, informed decision-making and personalized guidance are essential when considering the integration of the Fasting Mimicking Diet into one's lifestyle.

5.4: Religious and Cultural Fasting Practices

RELIGIOUS AND CULTURAL fasting practices have been observed for centuries and are deeply ingrained in the traditions and beliefs of many societies around the world. Fasting is a common practice in various religions such as Christianity, Islam, Judaism, Hinduism, Buddhism, and many others. These fasting traditions are often deeply rooted in religious texts, cultural customs, and communal practices, and they serve as a means of spiritual purification, self-discipline, and reflection. It is important to acknowledge and respect the diverse religious and cultural perspectives on fasting as we explore its various forms and interpretations.

In Christianity, fasting is often observed during Lent, which is a 40-day period of repentance, fasting, and preparation for Easter. Participants typically abstain from certain foods or activities as a way to reflect on the life and sacrifice of Jesus Christ. The Ramadan fast in Islam is one of the Five Pillars of Islam and is observed by Muslims worldwide. During the month of Ramadan, Muslims fast from dawn until sunset, refraining from eating, drinking, smoking, and engaging in sinful behavior. Fasting during Ramadan is viewed as an opportunity for selfdiscipline, empathy for the less fortunate, and spiritual reflection.

Judaism has several fasting days throughout the year, with Yom Kippur being the most significant. Yom Kippur, also known as the Day of Atonement, is observed with a 25-hour fast as a way to repent for sins and seek forgiveness from God. The Hindu tradition includes various fasting observances tied to religious festivals and special occasions. Fasting in Hinduism is believed to purify the body and mind and is often accompanied by prayers and rituals. Additionally, Buddhism has its own fasting practices, which can vary widely among different traditions and sects. Fasting is viewed as a way to develop mindfulness, discipline, and compassion towards all beings.

Other cultural and regional fasting practices exist around the world, often tied to specific rites of passage, agricultural cycles, or historical events. For example, some indigenous cultures have traditional fasting practices associated with healing rituals, initiation ceremonies, or communal gatherings. Similarly, fasting may play a role in traditional Chinese medicine and other holistic health practices.

Understanding the significance and practices of religious and cultural fasting can provide valuable insight into the deeper meaning and benefits of fasting beyond its physical effects. It is also important to recognize that fasting practices may not be suitable for everyone, and individuals should approach these traditions with respect and understanding of their cultural and spiritual significance.

By exploring the religious and cultural fasting practices of different societies, individuals can gain a broader appreciation for the diverse ways in which fasting is integrated into human experience and can find inspiration for incorporating fasting into their own health and wellness journeys. Appreciating these traditions can also foster empathy and understanding across different cultures and belief systems, enriching our collective appreciation for the profound impact of fasting on individuals and communities around the world.

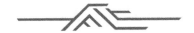

Chapter 6: Fasting for Longevity and Disease Prevention

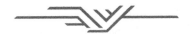

6.1: Fasting for Longevity

Fasting has been practiced for centuries for spiritual, cultural, and health reasons. In recent years, research has shown that fasting may have significant benefits for longevity. One of the key mechanisms through which fasting promotes longevity is autophagy, a process in which the body breaks down and recycles old or damaged cells. Autophagy is crucial for cellular health and has been linked to a reduced risk of age-related diseases such as cancer, neurodegenerative disorders, and cardiovascular disease.

According to a study published in Cell Metabolism, intermittent fasting has been shown to extend lifespan in mice by up to 30%. While more research is needed to fully understand the implications for humans, these findings are promising and suggest that fasting may play a role in promoting longevity. Another study published in the Journal of Nutrition, Health and Aging found that fasting may also help reduce inflammation, which is a key driver of aging and age-related diseases.

Fasting has also been associated with improvements in various biomarkers of aging and age-related diseases. For example, a study published in Rejuvenation

Research found that fasting can lead to reductions in insulin-like growth factor 1 (IGF-1) levels, a hormone that has been linked to aging and age-related diseases. Lower levels of IGF-1 have been associated with a reduced risk of cancer and increased longevity in animal studies.

In addition to its potential effects on aging and longevity, fasting has also been shown to have a profound impact on metabolic health. Multiple studies have demonstrated that fasting can improve insulin sensitivity, reduce blood pressure, and lower the risk of type 2 diabetes and heart disease. For example, a review article published in the New England Journal of Medicine concluded that intermittent fasting can lead to improvements in cardiovascular risk factors such as blood pressure, cholesterol levels, and markers of inflammation.

Furthermore, fasting has been shown to promote the production of brain-derived neurotrophic factor (BDNF), a protein that is essential for the growth, survival, and function of neurons. Higher levels of BDNF have been associated with a reduced risk of neurodegenerative diseases such as Alzheimer's and Parkinson's. In a study published in the Journal of Alzheimer's Disease, intermittent fasting was found to enhance cognitive function and have neuroprotective effects in animal models of Alzheimer's disease.

In conclusion, fasting has emerged as a promising strategy for promoting longevity and reducing the risk of age-related diseases. The scientific evidence supports the potential benefits of fasting for enhancing cellular health, improving metabolic parameters, and preserving cognitive function. While more research is needed to fully understand the long-term effects of fasting on human longevity, the existing findings suggest that incorporating fasting into a healthy lifestyle may offer significant advantages for promoting overall health and well-being.

6.2: Fasting and Chronic Disease Prevention

AS WE AGE, THE RISK of chronic diseases such as heart disease, diabetes, and cancer increases. Many studies have shown that fasting can play a significant role in preventing these diseases and promoting longevity. Fasting can help to reduce risk factors for chronic disease, such as inflammation, high blood pressure, high cholesterol, and insulin resistance.

One of the key benefits of fasting for chronic disease prevention is its impact on insulin sensitivity. Insulin resistance is a major risk factor for chronic diseases like type 2 diabetes and heart disease. Research has demonstrated that intermittent fasting can improve insulin sensitivity, lower fasting insulin levels, and reduce the risk of developing insulin resistance.

Moreover, fasting has been shown to have a positive impact on cardiovascular health. Studies have found that fasting can lead to improvements in blood pressure, cholesterol levels, and triglycerides, all of which are important markers for heart disease risk. For example, a study published in JAMA Internal Medicine in 2016 found that fasting interventions were associated with significant reductions in blood pressure, LDL cholesterol, and body mass index.

In addition to its effects on insulin sensitivity and cardiovascular health, fasting has also been linked to a reduced risk of cancer. Research in animal models has shown that fasting can slow the growth of tumors and enhance the effects of chemotherapy, while human studies have indicated that fasting may help protect against certain types of cancer. For example, a study published in the journal Science Translational Medicine in 2017 found that periodic fasting was associated with a lower risk of breast cancer recurrence in women who had been treated for early stage breast cancer.

Furthermore, fasting has been shown to reduce markers of inflammation, which is a key factor in the development of chronic diseases. Chronic inflammation has been linked to conditions such as arthritis, heart disease, and cancer. Studies have indicated that fasting can decrease levels of pro-inflammatory markers in the body, potentially reducing the risk of developing these conditions.

In conclusion, fasting has the potential to play a crucial role in preventing chronic diseases and promoting longevity. Its effects on insulin sensitivity, cardiovascular health, cancer risk, and inflammation make it a powerful tool for maintaining health as we age. By incorporating fasting into our lifestyles, we can work towards reducing the risk of chronic diseases and enjoying a longer, healthier life.

6.3: Fasting and Cellular Health

FASTING HAS SHOWN PROMISING potential for promoting cellular health, which is crucial for longevity and disease prevention. One of the key mechanisms through which fasting exerts its benefits is autophagy, a process in which the body cleans out damaged cells and regenerates new, healthy ones. Research has demonstrated that fasting can enhance autophagy, leading to improved cellular function and increased resistance to various chronic diseases. Studies have shown that intermittent fasting, in particular, can promote autophagy and reduce the risk of conditions such as cancer, Alzheimer's disease, and cardiovascular issues. For example, a study published in the journal Cell Research found that fasting activates autophagy in the brain, leading to a reduction in the accumulation of toxic proteins associated with neurodegenerative diseases. In addition, intermittent fasting has been shown to improve mitochondrial health, the powerhouses of our cells responsible for generating energy. By promoting mitochondrial biogenesis and function, fasting can enhance cellular energy production and reduce oxidative stress, thus supporting overall cellular health.

Furthermore, fasting can influence the activity of certain signaling pathways and genes that play a role in cellular protection and longevity. For instance, research has indicated that fasting activates sirtuins, a family of proteins that regulate cellular health and have been linked to longevity. Sirtuins are known to modulate various cellular processes, including DNA repair, inflammation, and stress response. By stimulating the activity of sirtuins, fasting may help protect cells from damage and contribute to overall resilience against age-related decline. Moreover, fasting has been shown to promote the expression of genes involved in antioxidant defense and DNA repair, offering further support for cellular health and resilience.

In addition to these molecular and cellular effects, fasting can also impact metabolic health, which is closely interconnected with cellular function. By improving insulin sensitivity and reducing inflammation, fasting can help mitigate metabolic dysfunction and its detrimental effects on cellular health. For example, research has demonstrated that intermittent fasting can lead to reductions in markers of systemic inflammation and improvements in insulin sensitivity, both of which are critical for maintaining healthy cells and tissues. By addressing these metabolic factors, fasting can contribute to the prevention of conditions such as type 2 diabetes, cardiovascular disease, and certain cancers, all of which significantly affect cellular health and contribute to the aging process.

Overall, the evidence suggests that fasting has the potential to profoundly impact cellular health, offering a powerful strategy for promoting longevity and preventing age-related diseases. By modulating autophagy, mitochondrial function, gene expression, and metabolic parameters, fasting can support the resilience and vitality of our cells, contributing to overall well-being and healthy aging. As we continue to uncover the intricate mechanisms through which fasting influences cellular health, it becomes increasingly clear that integrating fasting practices into our lifestyles may have far-reaching benefits for our longterm health and vitality.

6.4: Integrating Fasting into Healthy Aging

INCORPORATING FASTING into your lifestyle can play a profound role in healthy aging, providing a wide array of benefits for seniors looking to maintain their well-being and vitality as they age. Research has shown that fasting can have a positive impact on aging-related processes, including reducing inflammation, enhancing cellular repair, and promoting longevity. As we age, our bodies become more susceptible to chronic health conditions, such as cardiovascular disease, diabetes, and neurodegenerative disorders. Fasting has been demonstrated to offer protective effects against these age-related illnesses, making it a valuable tool for seniors striving to maintain their health.

One of the key mechanisms through which fasting contributes to healthy aging is through its ability to promote autophagy, the cellular process responsible for removing damaged components and maintaining cellular health. Autophagy is essential for prolonging the lifespan of cells, and fasting has been shown to stimulate this process, thereby contributing to improved cellular function and longevity. Moreover, fasting has been linked to enhanced cognitive function

and brain health in older adults. Studies have suggested that intermittent fasting may protect against age-related cognitive decline and reduce the risk of neurodegenerative diseases, such as Alzheimer's and Parkinson's disease.

Furthermore, integrating fasting into your lifestyle can have a significant impact on metabolic health, particularly for individuals in the senior age group. Fasting interventions, such as time-restricted feeding and periodic fasting, have been shown to improve insulin sensitivity, reduce blood sugar levels, and lower the risk of developing type 2 diabetes. Given that older adults are at a higher risk of experiencing metabolic disorders, these findings underscore the potential of fasting as a powerful strategy for mitigating age-related metabolic complications and promoting overall health.

In addition to the physiological benefits, fasting can also contribute to healthy aging by fostering a positive relationship with food and promoting mindful eating practices. By incorporating periods of fasting into your routine, you can develop a heightened awareness of hunger and satiety cues, ultimately leading to a more balanced and mindful approach to eating. This can be particularly beneficial for seniors seeking to maintain a healthy weight and prevent agerelated weight gain, which is associated with an increased risk of chronic diseases.

It's important to note that while fasting shows promise for healthy aging, it's crucial for seniors to consult with their healthcare providers before embarking on any fasting regimen. Medical supervision is particularly important for individuals with existing health conditions or those who are taking medications, as fasting may interact with certain medications or exacerbate underlying health issues. By working closely with a healthcare professional, seniors can tailor a fasting approach that aligns with their individual health needs and goals, ensuring a safe and effective integration of fasting into their lifestyle for optimal healthy aging.

Don't miss out!

Visit the website below and you can sign up to receive emails whenever Fasting Pioneer publishes a new book. There's no charge and no obligation.

https://books2read.com/r/B-A-DOZEB-NMMZC

BOOKS2READ

Connecting independent readers to independent writers.

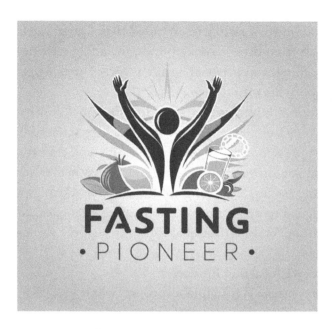

About the Author

About Fasting Pioneer

Welcome to the Fasting Pioneer author page, where the journey to health and well-being through the power of fasting begins. We are a collective of fasting enthusiasts with over a decade of personal and shared experiences in the fascinating world of fasting. Our passion lies not just in practicing fasting ourselves, but in sharing the wealth of knowledge we've accumulated over the years with people everywhere.

Our Mission At Fasting Pioneer, our mission is simple: to demystify the practice of fasting and make it accessible to everyone, regardless of their starting point. We believe in the transformative power of fasting to improve physical health, enhance mental clarity, and foster a deeper connection with one's body. Through our work, we aim to empower individuals to take control of their health and discover the profound benefits fasting can offer.

Our Expertise Over the last ten years, we've delved deep into the various facets of fasting, experimenting with and studying different methods, from intermittent fasting to extended fasts. Our group is composed of individuals from diverse backgrounds, including nutritional science, wellness coaching, and personal health advocacy, making our collective knowledge both broad and deep.

Our Contribution "Fasting for Health: The Ultimate Guide to Transform Your Life" represents the first in a long series of books about fasting. In it, we've poured all our insights, tips, and transformative stories to guide you on your own fasting journey. Whether you're curious about starting fasting or seeking to deepen your existing practice, our book is designed to be your companion, offering practical advice, scientific background, and motivational stories to support you every step of the way.

Connect with Fasting Pioneer:

Website: https://fastingpioneer.com/ Twitter (X): https://twitter.com/FastingPioneer

Read more at https://fastingpioneer.com/.

Printed in the USA
CPSIA information can be obtained
at www.ICGtesting.com
LVHW010418110724
785188LV00003B/258